HIV/AIDS

Hiv/Aids: Prevent It Then Also
Know How To Leave With It And
Have Your Work Well

Mary f. Phipps

Table of Contents

CHAPTER ONE

HIV AND HELPS

We integrate things we accept are useful for our perusers. We might get a little commission in the event that you make a buy through the connections on this page. Here is our method.

How we assess brands and items Helps is an illness that can strike HIV-positive people. Treatment with antiretroviral prescriptions can routinely hold Assists back from making in people with HIV.

HIV: What's going on here?

The HIV infection causes safe framework harm. HIV influences and kills CD4 cells a sort of resistant cell known as a Lymphocyte whenever left untreated.

The body is bound to foster different sicknesses and tumors over the long run as HIV kills more CD4 cells.

HIV is spread through the accompanying natural liquids:

- blood
- semen
- vaginal and rectal fluids
- chest milk

The disease isn't moved in air or water, or through nice contact.

Since HIV installs itself into the DNA of cells, it's a durable condition and at present there's no medicine that kills HIV from the body, though various scientists are endeavoring to consider one.

Notwithstanding, HIV can be overseen and lived with for a long time with the assistance of clinical consideration, including antiretroviral treatment.

AIDS, or Helps, is a difficult condition that can happen in HIV-positive individuals who don't get treatment.

The resistant framework is excessively powerless by then to

successfully battle different circumstances, contaminations, and infections.

As indicated by a dependable source, end-stage Helps patients with no treatment have a future of roughly three years. HIV can be overseen really with antiretroviral treatment, and future can be almost indistinguishable from that of a not contracted individual HIV.

1.2 million Americans are believed to be living with HIV right now. The fact that they have the infection makes one out of seven of those individuals ignorant.

The body can change because of HIV.

What is Helps

Helps is a disorder that can encourage in people with HIV. It is HIV's most developed stage. Nonetheless, HIV doesn't ensure that a singular will foster Guides.

HIV kills CD4 cells. CD4 counts normally range from 500 to 1,600 for each cubic millimeter in grown-ups who are solid. Helps will be analyzed in a HIV-positive individual whose CD4 count falls under 200 for every cubic millimeter.

In the event that an individual has HIV and fosters a pioneering contamination or malignant growth, which is phenomenal in non-HIV people, they may likewise be determined to have Helps.

Pneumocystis jiroveci pneumonia is an illustration of a deft disease that main influences seriously immunocompromised people, like those with cutting edge HIV contamination (Helps).

HIV can form into Helps in something like 10 years on the off chance that not treated. There's at present no solution for Helps, and without treatment, future subsequent to finding is about 3 years.

On the off chance that the individual gets a serious deft disease, this may be more limited. Nonetheless, antiretroviral treatment can prevent Helps from spreading.

Assuming Guides happens; it demonstrates that the invulnerable framework is seriously debilitated to where it can't successfully battle most of contaminations and sicknesses.

Thus, the individual living with Helps is bound to get various infections, **for example,**

- pneumonia
- Tuberculosis
- oral thrush, a parasitic condition in the mouth or throat
- cytomegalovirus (CMV), a kind of herpes contamination
- cryptococcal meningitis, a parasitic condition in the frontal cortex
- toxoplasmosis, a brain condition achieved by a parasite

- cryptosporidiosis, a condition achieved by a stomach related parasite
- infection, including Kaposi sarcoma (KS) and lymphoma

The condensed future associated with untreated Aides is positively not a quick result of the genuine problem. All things being equal, the illnesses and confusions accompany having a Guides debilitated safe framework.

HIV and Helps related complexities

The intense disease stage is the initial not many weeks after an individual agreements HIV. Early side effects of HIV

During this time, the contamination reproduces rapidly. HIV antibodies, which are proteins that go to lengths to safeguard against disease, are delivered by the singular's insusceptible framework as a reaction to the contamination.

During this stage, a few people at first display no side effects. In any case, numerous people experience aftereffects in the essential month or so directly following getting the contamination, yet they regularly don't comprehend HIV causes those secondary effects.

This is because of the way that intense stage side effects might look like those of influenza or other occasional infections.

They can go from gentle to serious, travel every which way, and last from a couple of days to a little while.

CHAPTER TWO

EARLY HIV SIDE EFFECTS

Fever, chills, enlarging of the lymph hubs, general a throbbing painfulness, a skin rash, a sensitive throat, a migraine, sickness, and a resentful stomach are side effects that are like those of normal diseases like influenza.

Furthermore, regardless of whether they, their primary care physician could imagine this season's virus or mononucleosis and not even HIV.

During this time, an individual's viral burden is very high, whether or not they show side effects. How much HIV in the circulation system is known as the viral burden?

HIV can without much of a stretch spread to others during this time span because of a high popular burden.

Beginning HIV secondary effects for the most part settle inside several months as the singular enters the progressing or clinical idleness, period of HIV. With treatment, this stage can keep going for quite a long time or even many years.

What are HIV's side effects?

HIV enters the clinical inactivity stage after vjbabout a month. From a couple of years to years and years, this stage can happen.

During this time, certain individuals have no side effects by any means, while others might have not many or no side effects by any stretch of the imagination. A side effect that isn't connected with a particular infection or condition is known as a vague side effect.

**Secondary effects could
include:**

- headaches and different a pounding excruciating quality
- extended lymph centers
- tedious fevers
- night sweats
- exhaustion
- affliction
- hurling
- free insides
- weight decrease
- skin rashes
- tedious oral or vaginal yeast sicknesses
- pneumonia
- shingles

Comparatively likewise with the starting stage, HIV is at this point versatile during this time even without secondary effects and can be conveyed to another person.

Be that as it may, except if an individual gets tried, they won't realize they have HIV. It is basic for an individual to get tried in the event that they show these side effects and accept they might have been presented to HIV.

As of now, HIV side effects could show up and go, or they could deteriorate rapidly. With treatment, this movement can be altogether dialed back.

Assuming therapy is begun adequately early, ongoing HIV can keep going for quite a long time with predictable utilization of this antiretroviral treatment and most likely won't advance to help.

Does rash show HIV?

The skin of numerous HIV-positive individuals' changes. Rash is every now and again one of the underlying indications of HIV contamination. More often than not, a HIV rash seems to be a lot of little, red, smoothed, raised spots.

HIV-related rashes HIV makes individuals bound to have skin issues on the grounds that the infection dispenses with insusceptible framework cells that battle contamination. Co-infections that can cause rash **include:**

Herpes simplex molluscum infectious shingles **the rash's still up in the air by:**

- what it resembles
- how long it perseveres
- how it might be managed depends upon the explanation

Rash associated with drug
While rash can be achieved by HIV co-infections, it can similarly be achieved by drug. A rash can be

brought about by certain drugs used to treat HIV or different circumstances.

In something like possibly 14 days of beginning another prescription, this sort of rash normally shows up. The rash may periodically disappear all alone. If it doesn't, a change of medications may be required.

An unfavorably susceptible response to drug can cause extreme rashes.

Different results of a horribly powerless reaction include: Stevens-Johnson disorder (SJS) is an intriguing unfavorably susceptible response to HIV drug that can incorporate difficulty breathing or gulping, unsteadiness, and fever. Fever and tongue and face enlarging are side effects. The rankling rash shows up rapidly and can influence the skin and mucous films.

Poisonous epidermal necrolysis, a possibly deadly condition that influences 30% of the skin, is known as the condition. Crisis clinical consideration is required in the event that this happens.

It's memorable's essential that rashes are normal and can be brought about by numerous different things, despite the fact that they can be brought about by HIV or HIV drugs.

Side effects of HIV in men: Is there a differentiation?

HIV side effects change from one individual to another; however people share large numbers of similar side effects. These side effects can show up and go, or they can deteriorate over the long haul.

An individual may likewise have been presented to other physically communicated infections (STIs) on the off chance that they have been presented to HIV. These include:

Trichomoniasis, gonorrhea, chlamydia, syphilis, and gonorrhea might be more normal in men and those with a penis to see genital bruises as STI side effects than in ladies. Notwithstanding, men are more outlandish than ladies to look for clinical consideration.

CHAPTER THREE

MEN'S HIV SIDE EFFECTS

Side effects of HIV in ladies:

HIV side effects are by and large similar in people. Notwithstanding, because of the various dangers people face when they have HIV, their general side effects might contrast.

HIV-positive people are bound to contract STIs. Nonetheless, it's conceivable that ladies and the people who have a vagina are more outlandish than men to see any modifications or little spots in their private parts.

Furthermore, HIV-positive ladies are bound to experience the **ill effects of:**

intermittent vaginal yeast contaminations other vaginal diseases, for example, bacterial vaginosis pelvic incendiary sickness (PID) feminine cycle changes human papillomavirus (HPV), which can make genital moles and lead cervical malignant growth. Albeit this hazard isn't connected with the side effects of HIV, ladies who have the infection risked giving it to their unborn youngster during pregnancy. In any case, antiretroviral treatment is seen as safeguarded during pregnancy.

Antiretroviral treatment lessens the probability of a lady passing HIV to her unborn kid during pregnancy and conveyance. HIV-positive ladies likewise dislike breastfeeding. The disease can be moved to a kid through chest milk.

In the US and various settings where recipe is open and safe, it's recommended that women with HIV not breastfeed their kids. Equation use is empowered for these ladies.

Sanitized human milk is an option in contrast to recipe.

Fundamental for ladies might have been presented to HIV to know about the side effects to search for.

Figure out more about ladies' HIV side effects.

Results of Helps

AIDS is alluded to as Helps. With this condition, the protected system is weakened as a result of HIV that is ordinarily gone untreated for quite a while.

If HIV is found and treated exactly on schedule with antiretroviral therapy, a singular will normally not cultivate Guides.

Assuming they know that they have HIV yet don't in every case take their antiretroviral treatment, HIV-positive people risk creating Helps.

Assuming that they have a type of HIV that is impervious to (doesn't answer) antiretroviral treatment, they risk creating Helps too.

HIV-positive individuals might foster Guides prior on the off chance that they don't get steady and compelling treatment. By that point, the safe framework is seriously compromised and makes some harder memories answering ailment and contamination.

With the use of antiretroviral treatment, an individual can keep a tenacious HIV assurance without making Helps for a seriously lengthy timespan.

Helps related side effects can include:

Intermittent or ongoing looseness of the bowels fast weight reduction neurologic issues like difficulty concentrating, cognitive decline, and disarray uneasiness and despondency antiretroviral treatment control the infection and generally forestall movement to Helps. Ongoing enlarged lymph organs, particularly those in the armpits, neck, and crotch. ongoing weakness. Dull splotches under the skin or inside the mouth, nose, or eyelids. Helps related intricacies and different contaminations can likewise be dealt with. That treatment should be custom-made to the individual's particular prerequisites.

HIV transmission real factors
Anyone can contract HIV. The infection is spread through natural **liquids like:**

- Blood, sperm, vaginal and rectal liquids, and bosom milk are wellsprings of HIV transmission.

- through vaginal or butt-driven sex the most generally perceived course of transmission
- by sharing needles, needles, and various things for implantation drug use
- by sharing tattoo equipment without sanitizing it between uses
- during pregnancy, work, or transport from a pregnant person to their youngster
- during breastfeeding
- through "premastication," or gnawing a youngster's

food preceding dealing with it to them

- through receptiveness to the blood, semen, vaginal and rectal fluids, and chest milk of someone living with HIV, for instance, through a needle stick

The disease can similarly be conveyed through a blood holding or organ and tissue move. Nonetheless, this is very exceptional in the US because of thorough HIV testing of blood, organ, and tissue givers.

HIV could hypothetically be communicated through; however this is viewed as **incredibly impossible:**

- Oral sex (given that there are depleting gums or open injuries in the singular's mouth)
- being sacked by a person with HIV (given that the spit is absurd or there are open injuries in the singular's mouth)
- contact between broken skin, wounds, or mucous movies and the blood of someone living with HIV

HIV doesn't travel through: skin-to-skin contact; kissing, embracing, or shaking hands; sharing air or water; sharing food or beverages, including wellsprings; sharing spit, tears, or sweat (except if blended in with HIV blood); sharing a latrine; towels; or then again bedding; mosquitoes or different bugs. It is crucial for note that it is basically unimaginable for an individual living with HIV to send the infection to someone else assuming that they are getting treatment and have a viral burden that is steadily imperceptible.

Get more to know HIV transmission.

HIV is an infection that can be given to African chimpanzees through a variety. At the point when people consumed chimpanzee meat containing the simian immunodeficiency infection (SIV), researchers accept the infection spread from chimps to people.

The infection changed into HIV once it entered the human populace. This most probable occurred during the 1920s.

HIV spread starting with one individual then onto the next all through Africa all through an extremely extended period of time. Finally, the contamination moved to various region of the planet. In 1959, researchers tracked down HIV without precedent for an example of human blood.

It's accepted that HIV has existed in the US since the 1970s, yet it didn't start to hit public mindfulness until the 1980s.

Get more familiar with the American history of HIV and Helps.

CHAPTER FOUR

TREATMENT DECISIONS
FOR HIV

Treatment should begin as fast as far as possible after a finish of HIV, paying little psyche to viral weight.

The important treatment for HIV is antiretroviral treatment, a blend of ordinary medications that keep the disease from reproducing. By safeguarding CD4 cells, the resistant framework stays sufficiently able to ward off illness.

Antiretroviral treatment helps keep HIV away from progressing to Help. Furthermore, it supports bringing down the gamble of HIV disease to other people.

The viral burden will be "imperceptible" when treatment is fruitful. The individual keeps on having HIV; however the infection isn't obvious in that frame of mind of the tests.

Notwithstanding, the body actually contains the infection. Yet again also, if that singular suspends antiretroviral treatment, the viral burden will increment again, permitting HIV to start going after CD4 cells.

HIV medicines there are various endorsed antiretroviral treatment medicines. They work to prevent HIV from duplicating and eliminating CD4 cells, which help the safe framework in battling disease.

Both the gamble of contracting HIV entanglements and the probability of giving the infection to others are decreased thus.

**Seven classes of these
antiretroviral drugs:**

Non-nucleoside turn around transcriptase inhibitors (NNRTIs), protease inhibitors, combination inhibitors, and nucleoside invert transcriptase inhibitors

Treatment regimens The US Division of Wellbeing and Human Administrations (HHS) by and large suggest a beginning routine of three HIV prescriptions from no less than two of these medication classes. CCR5 adversaries are otherwise called passage inhibitors; integrate strand move inhibitors, and connection inhibitors.

HIV is kept from creating drug opposition on account of this mix. Obstruction demonstrates that the medication never again really battles the infection.)

Since a considerable lot of the antiretroviral drugs are joined with others, HIV patients normally just require a couple of pills each day.

A clinical benefits provider will help a person with HIV pick an everyday practice considering their overall prosperity and individual circumstances.

These prescriptions should be required as coordinated consistently. Viral opposition might create on the off chance that they are not taken as coordinated, requiring another treatment plan.

Blood testing will assist with concluding whether the routine is endeavoring to hold the viral weight down and the CD4 count up. If an antiretroviral therapy routine isn't working, the singular's clinical consideration provider will transform them to another schedule that is really convincing.

Expenses and aftereffects antiretroviral treatment can cause different secondary effects, including queasiness, cerebral pain, and unsteadiness. These side effects habitually last just a brief time frame and reduce over the long haul.

Expanding of the tongue and mouth as well as harm to the liver or kidney is serious incidental effects. The meds can be adjusted in light of serious aftereffects.

The expense of antiretroviral treatment changes relying upon where you reside and what sort of protection you have. A couple of medication associations have assist undertakings to help with cutting down the cost.

HIV and AIDS: Is there a connection?

An individual high priority contracted HIV to foster Guides. However, having HIV doesn't be ensured to infer that someone will cultivate Guides.

HIV cases go through three phases:

Stage 1: intense stage, the initial not many weeks following

Stage 2 transmission: ongoing stage

Stage 3: clinical inertness HIV debilitates the safe framework as the quantity of CD4 cells diminishes. The CD4 count of a typical grown-up is somewhere in the range of 500 and 1,500 for each cubic millimeter. A person with a count under 200 is considered to have Makes a difference.

How quickly an occurrence of HIV propels through the continuous stage changes basically starting with one individual then onto the next. It can endure as long as 10 years without treatment prior to advancing to Help. It can keep going for quite a long time with treatment.

There's at present no answer for HIV, yet it will in general be made due. At the point when HIV is dealt with right on time with antiretroviral treatment, a great many people carry on with a typical life expectancy.

Additionally, there is at present no known treatment for Helps. In any case, treatment can make the most of an individual's CD4 high to such an extent that they are not generally considered to have Helps. A count of 200 or higher demonstrates this point.)

Also, treatment can ordinarily help with directing insightful illnesses.

In spite of the fact that they are connected, HIV and Helps isn't exactly the same thing.

Figure out additional about the qualifications among Helps and HIV.

HIV is the infection that causes Helps. Without having contracted HIV, an individual can't contract Helps.

CD4 counts range from 500 to 1,500 for every cubic millimeter in solid people. HIV proceeds to spread and annihilate CD4 cells without treatment. An individual has Helps in the event that their CD4 count is fewer than 200.

Likewise, regardless of whether an individual's CD4 count is over 200, they can in any case be determined to have Helps in the event that they get a pioneering disease that is connected to HIV.

CHAPTER SIX

SORTS OF TESTS USED TO PRECLUDE HIV

A couple of particular tests can be used to break down HIV. Clinical benefits providers sort out which test is best for each person.

The most often utilized tests are neutralizer/antigen tests. They can show positive results regularly inside 18-45 days after someone at first arrangements HIV.

These tests search for antibodies and antigens in the blood. An immunizer is a kind of protein the body makes to answer defilement. An antigen, on the other hand, is the piece of the contamination that authorizes the insusceptible system.

Immunizer tests

These tests check the blood solely for antibodies. A great many people will foster HIV antibodies that can be identified in their blood or spit somewhere in the range of 23 and 90 days subsequent to being uncovered.

These tests are done using blood tests or mouth swabs, and there's no availability basic. A few tests can be acted in a medical care supplier's office or facility and give results in less than 30 minutes.

Other locally established immunizer tests include: HIV OraQuick Experimental outcomes can be acquired in just 20 minutes with an oral swab.

Framework for HIV-1 testing at home: After the singular pricks their finger, they send a blood test to an approved examination community. They can remain obscure and call for results the accompanying work day.

On the off chance that an individual accepts they have been presented to HIV yet gets an adverse outcome from a home test, they ought to have the test retaken in three months or less. In case they have a positive result, they should return again to their clinical consideration provider to certify.

Nucleic analysis (NAT): This exorbitant test isn't utilized for separating general. It is expected for people with HIV's initial side effects or a realized gamble factor. Antibodies are not the focal point of this test; it looks for the infection in general.

HIV can be identified in the blood somewhere in the range of 5 to 21 days after contamination. Normally, an immune response test is finished related to or to affirm this test.

Today, it's clearer than any time in late memory to get pursued for HIV.

How long is the HIV window? At the point when someone contracts HIV, it starts to rehash in their body. The individual's resistant framework produces antibodies in light of the antigens parts of the infection by going to antiviral lengths.

The time between receptiveness to HIV and when it becomes recognizable in the blood is known as the HIV window period. Inside

23 to 90 days of being tainted, most of individuals foster HIV antibodies that can be identified.

Almost certainly, an individual will get an adverse outcome from a HIV test on the off chance that they take it during the window. Regardless, they can anyway send the disease to others during this time.

On the off chance that an individual accepts they might have been presented to HIV yet didn't test positive at that point, they ought to step through the exam again in a couple of months to affirm (the timing relies upon the test). Moreover, they should utilize condoms or other boundary techniques during that opportunity to forestall HIV transmission.

Post-openness prophylaxis (Enthusiasm) might be gainful for somebody who tests negative during the window. This is remedy taken after receptiveness to thwart getting HIV.

After the openness, Energy should be taken quickly; it ought to be required inside the initial 72 hours of openness, yet at the same preferably prior.

Another technique for thwarting getting HIV is pre-receptiveness prophylaxis (PrEP). When taken reliably, PrEP, a mix of HIV prescriptions taken before potential HIV openness, can bring down the gamble of contracting or sending HIV.

Timing is critical while testing for HIV.

How HIV test results are impacted by timing.

HIV avoidance regardless of the endeavors of various analysts, there is at present no immunization to forestall HIV transmission. In any case, there are steps that can help with forestalling HIV transmission.

More secure sex without a condom or other boundary, butt-centric or vaginal sex is the most well-known technique for HIV transmission. This chance can't be totally disposed of without keeping away from sex, yet by avoiding potential risk, it tends to be essentially diminished.

An individual who is stressed over their HIV hazard ought to:

Get pursued for HIV. They should know about both their own and their accomplice's status.

Get checked for some other STIs (physically sent infections). They ought to look for treatment in the event that they test positive for one, as having a STI improves the probability of contracting HIV.

Use condoms. They should get to know the right technique for using condoms and use them each time they have sex, whether it's through vaginal or butt-driven intercourse. Remember that pre-fundamental liquids, which are delivered before male discharge, may contain HIV.

In the event that they have HIV, accept their meds as coordinated. Accordingly, they are more averse

to spread the infection to their
accomplice.

CHAPTER SIX

DIFFERENT MEANS TO FORESTALL HIV SPREAD

Different method for forestalling the spread of HIV incorporates the accompanying **extra measures:**

Make an effort not to share needles or other stuff. HIV is sent through blood and can be contracted by using materials that have associated with the blood of someone who has HIV.

Ponder Kick: Assuming you've been presented to HIV, you ought to converse with your PCP about getting post-openness prophylaxis (Enthusiasm). HIV contamination hazard can be lower with Kick. It comprises of three 28-day courses of antiretroviral medicine.

After openness, Energy ought to be started at the earliest opportunity, however no later than 36 to 72 hours after the fact.

Contemplate PrEP: Pre-openness prophylaxis, or PrEP, ought to be examined with a medical services supplier on the off chance that an individual has a higher gamble of contracting HIV. It might bring down HIV disease risk when taken routinely. The mix of two prescriptions referred to as Prepare is accessible as a pill.

More insights concerning these and alternate ways of preventing HIV from spreading can be given by medical services experts.

Living with HIV: What the future holds and ways of adjusting

More than 1.2 million people in the US are living with HIV. It shifts from one individual to another, yet many individuals can expect a long and useful existence with treatment.

Beginning antiretroviral treatment as quickly as time permits is really significant. Individuals with HIV can keep their viral burden low and their invulnerable framework solid by accepting their drugs as coordinated.

It's in like manner crucial to return again to a clinical consideration provider reliably.

Alternate ways HIV-positive individuals can further develop their **wellbeing are:**

Focus on their wellbeing regardless of anything else. Pushes toward help with peopling living with HIV feel their **best include:**

- filling their body with an in any event, eating schedule
- rehearsing regularly

- getting a great deal of rest
- avoiding tobacco and various meds
- uncovering any new aftereffects to their clinical consideration provider right away
- Revolve around their mental wellbeing. They could contemplate seeing an authorized specialist who has experience treating HIV patients.

Utilize more secure techniques for sex. Connect with their expected sexual accomplices. Get pursued for other STIs. What's more, at whatever point they have butt-centric or vaginal sex, they ought to utilize condoms and other obstruction strategies.

Talk about PrEP and Kick with their medical services supplier. Pre-openness prophylaxis (PrEP) and post-openness prophylaxis (Enthusiasm) can bring down the probability of transmission when utilized reliably by a sans hiv person. In associations with HIV-positive individuals, PrEP is commonly suggested; however it can likewise be utilized in different circumstances. Online focal points for finding a PrEP provider consolidate PrEP Locater and PleasePrEPMe.

Assemble with friends and family around them. At the point when individuals are first told about their determination, they can begin gradually by let somebody know who can keep them sure. They could have to pick someone who won't condemn them and who will maintain them in zeroing in on their prosperity.

Get some assistance: They can meet with other people who are managing similar issues as they are by joining a HIV support bunch, either face to face or on the web. Furthermore, their medical services supplier can guide them to different neighborhood assets.

While living with HIV, there are various procedures for boosting personal satisfaction.

Advance a few genuine stories from HIV-positive people.

Future for HIV: Know current realities: A 20-year-old with HIV had a 19-year future during the 1990s, as per a confided in source. By 2011, a 20-year-old person with HIV could expect to encounter 53 extra years.

It is a critical improvement, generally due to antiretroviral treatment. Numerous HIV patients can carry on with typical or close typical lives with appropriate treatment.

Clearly, various things impact future for a person with HIV. **Some of them are:**

CD4 cell count viral burden serious HIV-related ailments like hepatitis, illicit drug use, smoking, admittance to treatment, and reaction to treatment for other medical issue age People in the US and other made countries may will undoubtedly approach antiretroviral therapy.

Taking these meds consistently helps prevent HIV from transforming into Helps. As indicated by a solid source, the future without treatment for HIV/Helps is roughly three years.

Antiretroviral treatment was involved by roughly 20.9 million HIV-positive people in 2017.

Insights about future are simply common rules. To more deeply study what's in store, HIV-positive individuals ought to converse with their PCP or medical attendant.

CHAPTER SEVEN

VACCINATION FOR HIV

There is right now no HIV antibodies or medicines. Exploratory immunizations are the subject of progressing examination and testing, however none are near being supported for broad use.

The HIV infection is convoluted. It transforms (changes) quickly and every now and again opposes reactions from the resistant framework. Comprehensively killing antibodies, which are antibodies that are fit for answering an assortment of HIV strains, are just created by a little level of HIV-positive people.

2016 saw the beginning of the first HIV immunization viability concentrate in quite a while in South Africa. The exploratory immunization is a later variant of one that was tried in a 2009 Thai preliminary.

A 3.5-year drag along vaccination showed the inoculation was 31.2 percent strong in thwarting HIV transmission.

5,400 South African people are remembered for the review. In South Africa, roughly 270,000 individuals contracted HIV in

2016. The review's discoveries are expected in 2021.

Other late-stage, worldwide vaccination clinical fundamentals are moreover underway.

An immunization against HIV is likewise the subject of continuous examination.

While there's still no inoculation to thwart HIV, people with HIV can benefit from various antibodies to hinder HIV-related sicknesses. **The CDC suggests the accompanying:**

Pneumonia: suggested for all young people more energetic than

2 and generally adults 65 and more settled

Influenza: suggested for all people in excess of a half year old yearly with extraordinary unique cases

Hepatitis A and B: Inquire as to whether you ought to get immunization against hepatitis An and B, especially in the event that you have a place with a gathering at higher gamble. As per Confided in Source, the meningococcal form immunization is suggested for all youngsters and teenagers between the ages of 11 and 12, with a promoter portion given at 16 for the people who are in danger. Anybody beyond 10 a years old is at an expanded gamble ought to receive an immunization shot against serogroup B meningococcal sickness.

Shingles: suggested A legitimate hotspot for individuals 50 and more seasoned Realize the reason why fostering a HIV immunization is so difficult.

HIV measurements

HIV impacted roughly 38 million individuals overall in 2019. 1.8 million Of those were kids younger than 15.

Toward the finish of 2019, antiretroviral treatment was being utilized by 25.4 million HIV-positive people.

75.7 million Individuals have contracted HIV since the pandemic started, and 32.7 million individuals have kicked the bucket because of Helps related inconveniences.

690,000 individuals passed on from Helps related sicknesses in 2019. This is lower than the 2005 figure of 1.9 million.

The most impacted districts are Eastern and Southern Africa. In these districts, 20.7 million individuals were tainted with HIV in 2019 and another 730,000 gotten the infection. The greater part of the world's HIV-positive populace lives around here.

In 2018, grown-up and juvenile ladies contained 19% of new HIV analyze in the US. Near portion of all new cases occur in African Americans.

A lady with HIV has a 15-45% possibility passing the infection to her child while she is pregnant or breastfeeding in the event that she doesn't seek treatment. The gamble is under 5% with antiretroviral treatment all through pregnancy and breastfeeding precluded, as per Confided in Source.

A 20-year-old with HIV had a Confided in Source future of 19 years during the 1990s. It had improved to 53 years by 2011. In the event that antiretroviral treatment is begun not long after contracting HIV, future today is near typical, as per confided in sources. These figures, it is trusted, will keep on fluctuating as worldwide admittance to antiretroviral treatment gets to the next level.

www.ingramcontent.com/pod-product-compliance
Lightning Source LLC
Chambersburg PA
CBHW051835250726
48659CB00005B/1845